Skincare Starts with Self-Care

Niccol A

Copyright © 2024 Niccol A

All rights reserved.

ISBN: 9798323124770

i

DEDICATION

To my husband "Ron" that pushes me daily, keeps me encouraged and gives those forehead kisses when I've had a long day. To my father "Jimmy", who never stopped believing in me. To my daughters, Chyynnah and Nikole who are my walking heartbeats. To my friend "Demitri" who continued to believe in me when I didn't believe in myself and prays for and with me daily. To my Pastor Rev. Dr. Frankco Harris of Mt. Olivet Baptist Church of Hollis, Queens who told me that I have a gift, to spread my wings and reminds me, when I fell discouraged that "I can do all things through Christ that Strengthens me". To you, my dear readers for making this journey worthwhile. To the younger me that wouldn't be quiet and always had a million questions, keep talking and keep learning. To the countless influencers I sat and binge watched daily, thank you. "50 Cent" aka Curtis Jackson for getting me through that 3 year walk down. To the past that made me, the present that nurtures me and the future that awaits me. To GOD, for guiding my journey.

CONTENTS

PRETTI PLEASE BEAUTY CO.

SKIN CARE STARTS WITH SELF-CARE:

A Comprehensive Guide to Nourishing Your Skin and Soul

1 INTRODUCTION: THE IMPORTANCE OF SELF-CARE

In our fast-paced world, it's easy to neglect ourselves amidst the hustle and bustle of everyday daily life. Life just be lifing right? However, self-care isn't just a luxury- it's a necessity. This book will guide you through the journey of nurturing your skin and soul, helping you achieve a state of radiance from within.

In this chapter, we'll delve into why self-care is essential and why you'll any to keep turning the pages to discover how it can transform your life.

Why self-care matters:

Let's be honest, life can get hectic. Between work, family responsibilities, the endless stream of notifications on our phones and staying up to date in all celebrity drama. It's easy to feel overwhelmed and burnt out. But here's the truth: Self-Care isn't selfish; it's a necessary. Just like you need to recharge your phone to keep it running smoothly, you need to recharge yourself to show up as your best self in all aspects of your life.

The ripple effect: How self-care impacts every area of your life:

You might be thinking, "But I don't have time for self-care". Trust us, we get it. But here's the thing: when you prioritize self-care, you're not just taking care of yourself – you're investing in your relationships, your work, and your overall well-being. When you feel good, you're better equipped to handle whatever life throws your way. So by taking care of yourself, you're actually setting yourself up for success in every area of your life.

Why you'll want to keep reading:

So why should you keep reading? Because Pretti, we're about to show you how to incorporate self-care into your daily routine in a way that's simple, practical, and most importantly, sustainable. Whether you're a skincare novice or a self-care enthusiast, this book has something for everyone. From skincare tips to stress management techniques, we've got you covered.

Get ready to transform your life:

Are you ready to say goodbye to stress, dull skin, and burnout? Are you ready to say hello to glowing skin, inner peace, and a renewed sense of vitality? Then keep reading, because **Pretti Please Beauty Co.** is about to become your go-to guide for transforming your life-one self-care practice at a time.

Get ready to embark on a journey of self-discovery and self-love. Get ready to prioritize yourself in a world that often tells you to put everyone else first. A world where you pour and pour and pour into everything and everyone else but your left dry, thirsty and dehydrated. Get ready to drink and embrace your glow, inside and out.

**WELCOME TO THE PRETTI SQUAD!
YOU HAVE FOUND YOUR TRIBE**

**Philippians 4:13
I Can Do All Things Through Christ That Strengthens Me!**

2 UNDERSTANDING YOUR SKIN: YOUR UNIQUE CANVAS

Welcome to the canvas of you! We're about to dive deep into the world of skincare. Where your skin takes center stage as the star of the show. Get ready to embark on a journey of self discovery as we explore the fascinating landscape of skin types and what makes yours uniquely beautiful.

Your skin: A marvelous Mosaic of Diversity

Just like a fingerprint, your skin is one of a kind. From the smoothest porcelain to the richest cocoa, skin comes in a stunning array of shades, the tires and tones. Whether you're fair-skinned with freckles or blessed with a luminous melanin-rich complexion, your skin tells a story of your heritage, your lifestyle, and your journey through life. Welcome to the world of skincare , where every complexion tells a unique story. Whether you're a fair-skinned beauty or blessed with a sun-kissed glow, your skin deserves to be celebrated and pampered. In this chapter we'll explore the diverse landscape of skin types, common frustrations faced by individuals with a multitude of skin pigmentations, and empowering solutions to help you achieve your skincare goals.

The skin you're in: Embracing your unique features

Forget about airbrushed perfection – Real Beauty lies in embracing your unique features. Maybe you've got a smattering of cute little moles that dance across your cheeks like constellations in the night sky. Perhaps you've got laugh lines that tell tales of joyous moments shared with loved ones. Whatever quirks and characteristics make your skin uniquely yours, Pretti, TODAY your going to learn to celebrate them with pride!

Decoding your skin type detective 👀

Are you a slick superhero with oil-prone skin? A desert oasis in need of hydration? Or perhaps you're a balanced beauty who's got it all figured out. No matter your skin type, understanding its unique needs is the first step towards achieving a radiant glowing complexion. Get ready to channel your inner skin detective as we decode the clues your skin is giving you and uncover the secrets to a happy, healthy, glowing complexion.

Skin Type Hinting Expedition: Exploring The Complexities of Your Skin:

Join us on a hunt through the wilderness of skin types as we encounter oily oases, dry deserts, combination continents, and sensitive sanctuaries. From the thrill of discovery to the satisfaction of finding your skins perfect match, this journey promises to be as exhilarating as it is enlightening.

Why you'll love this chapter:

Get ready to fall in love with your skin all over again! This chapter isn't just about identifying your skin type - it's about celebrating the skin you're in and learning how to give it the love and care it deserves. With fun, interactive quizzes, helpful tips, and plenty of surprises along the way, this chapter promises to be an adventure you won't want to miss!

So grab your magnifying glass and your explorer's hat, because we're about to embark on a thrilling expedition adventure though the marvelous world of your skin!

Discover Your Skin Type: The Ultimate Skincare Adventure

Embark on a thrilling skincare adventure as we uncover the mysteries of your skin type. Take our interactive quiz to identify your unique skin profile and unlock personalized tips and tricks for achieving a radiant complexion. From oily oases to dry deserts, find out which skincare landscape you call home and how to navigate it with confidence.

The many Skin Types for FAIR SKIN Individuals:

- **Your Normal Navigators:** Blessed with balanced skin that's neither too oily nor too dry, Normal Navigators enjoy smooth sailing on their skincare journey.

- **Oily Oasis Explorers:** For those who struggle with excess oil production, navigating the Oily Oasis can be a challenge. But fear not—we've got solutions to keep shine at bay and your complexion looking fresh.

- **Dry Desert Dwellers:** Desert-dry skin can leave you feeling parched and in need of hydration. Explore tips and tricks to quench your skin's thirst and restore moisture balance.

- **Combination Continent Adventurers:** Balancing act got you feeling like a tightrope walker? Join the ranks of Combination Continent Adventurers as we explore strategies for managing both oily and dry zones.

- **Sensitive Sanctuary Seekers:** Sensitivity can turn skincare into a minefield, but with the right approach, you can create a soothing sanctuary for your delicate skin.

- **Acne-Prone Pathfinders:** Bumps, blemishes, and breakouts—oh my! Acne-Prone Pathfinders face a rocky road, but with targeted treatments, clear skin is within reach.

- **Sun-Sensitive Voyagers:** Sun exposure can leave your skin feeling fried and frazzled. Discover how to protect your skin from harmful UV rays and prevent sun damage.

- **Redness-Prone Pilgrims:** Rosy cheeks are charming, but persistent redness can be frustrating. Learn how to calm inflammation and reduce redness for a more even complexion.

- **Fine Line Explorers:** Time may be on your side, but fine lines and wrinkles are not. Explore anti-aging strategies to keep your skin looking youthful and vibrant.

- **Dullness Dwellers:** Lackluster skin got you feeling blah? Brighten up with tips and tricks to restore radiance and unveil your natural glow

Now Lets discuss your top Skin Frustrations but with some Solutions:

- **Frustration:** Excess oiliness.
- **Solution:** Incorporate oil-balancing cleansers and lightweight moisturizers into your routine.

- **Frustration:** Dry, flaky skin.
- **Solution:** Hydrate from within by drinking plenty of water and using rich, emollient moisturizers.

- **Frustration:** Breakouts and acne.
- **Solution:** Treat acne-prone areas with gentle, non-comedogenic products containing ingredients like salicylic acid or benzoyl peroxide.

- **Frustration:** Sunburn and sun damage.
- **Solution:** Protect your skin with broad-spectrum sunscreen and seek shade during peak sun hours.

- **Frustration:** Redness and irritation.

- **Solution**: Use soothing ingredients like aloe vera and chamomile to calm inflammation and reduce redness.

- **Frustration**: Fine lines and wrinkles.
- **Solution**: Incorporate retinoids and antioxidants into your skincare routine to promote collagen production and combat signs of aging..

- **Frustration**: Dull, lackluster skin.
- **Solution**: Exfoliate regularly to remove dead skin cells and reveal a brighter, more radiant complexion

- **Frustration**: Sensitivity and irritation
- **Solution**: Opt for fragrance-free, hypoallergenic products formulated for sensitive skin.

- **Frustration**: Uneven skin tone and dark spots.
- **Solution**: Incorporate brightening ingredients like vitamin d C and NIACIN-AMIDE into your skincare routine to fade discoloration and promote an even complexion.

- **Frustration**: Enlarged pores and rough texture.
- **Solution**: Use gentle exfoliants and pore-minimizing serums to refine skin texture and reduce the appearance of pores.

Let's Discuss Embracing Your Beautiful Darker Melanin Skin:

Welcome to a celebration of beautiful, glowing skin! Lets dive in and explore the diverse world of darker melanin skincare, from the rich hues of melanin to the unique challenges faced by individuals with darker skin tones. Get ready to embark on a journey of self-discovery as we uncover your skin type, address common frustrations, and unlock the secrets to a glowing complexion.

Hey Pretti, Let's Discover Your Skin Type:

Your skin is as unique as you are, and understanding its type is the key to unlocking its full potential. Take our interactive quiz to uncover your skin's true essence and receive personalized tips and recommendations to enhance your natural beauty. Whether you're blessed with supple cocoa butter skin or navigating the complexities of combination skin, we're here to guide you on your journey to radiant skin.

The top skin types for AFRICAN AMERICAN individuals:

- **Melanin Majesty:** Bask in the glory of your melanin-rich complexion, which offers natural protection against UV damage and premature aging.

- **Oily Oasis:** Navigate the challenges of excess oil production, which can lead to shine and breakouts, especially in the T-zone.

- **Dry Desert:** Experience the thirst of dry skin, often exacerbated by harsh weather conditions and environmental factors.

- **Combination Conundrum:** Struggle with the dual nature of combination skin, with an oily T-zone and dry cheeks requiring different care.

- **Sensitive Sanctuary:** Seek solace for sensitive skin, prone to irritation and inflammation, especially when exposed to harsh chemicals or fragrances.

- **Acne-Prone Pioneer:** Brave the battlefield of acne-prone skin, where blemishes and breakouts can leave scars and dark spots behind.

- **Hyperpigmentation Hero:** Conquer the challenge of hyperpigmentation, which can manifest as dark spots, patches, or uneven skin tone.

- **Ashy Anomaly:** Combat the common complaint of ashy skin, caused by a lack of moisture and hydration, particularly in colder climates.

- **Keloid Kingdom:** Rule over the realm of keloids, where raised scars can develop after injury or inflammation, requiring specialized care.

- **Elasticity Empire:** Preserve the elasticity and firmness of your skin, which may be prone to sagging and loss of definition over time.

Skin Type Quiz: Discover Your Skin's Unique Needs

Take this quick quiz to determine your skin type and unlock personalized skincare recommendations tailored to your specific concerns and goals.

1.HOW DOES YOUR SKIN FEEL AFTER CLEANSING?

A) Tight and dry

B) Clean and comfortable

C) Oily or greasy

2. Throughout the day, how does your skin appear?

A) Dull and lackluster

B) Balanced and healthy-looking

C) Shiny or oily

3. Don't experience and tightness or discomfort after applying skincare products?

A) Yes, often

B) Occasionally

C) Rarely or never

4. How does your skin react to new skincare products?

A) It tends to feel sensitive or irritated

B) It adapts well without any adverse reactions

C) It may become more oily or breakout – prone

5. Do you notice any visible pores on your skin?

A) Yes, they're small and barely noticeable

B) Yes, they're visible but not enlarged

C) Yes, they're large and prominent

6. How does your skin feel by the end of the day?

A) Tight and dry

B) Comfortable and balanced

C) Oily or greasy

Results:

Mostly A's: Your skin type may be dry/dehydrated. Your skin tends to feel tight and dry. Especially after cleansing, and may appear dull or lackluster. It's important to focus on hydrating and nourishing your skin with rich moisturizers and hydrating serums.

Mostly B's: Your skin type may be normal/combination. Your skin is generally well-balanced, with minimal concerns and few visible imperfections. Maintain your skin's equilibrium with a balanced skincare routine that addresses any occasional dryness or oiliness.

Mostly C's: Your skin type may be oily/acne-prone. Your skin tends to produce excess oil, leading to a shiny or greasy appearance throughout the day. Focus on balancing oil production with lightweight, non-comedogenic products and targeted treatments for acne-prone skin.

No matter your skin type, remember to listen to your skins needs and adjust your skin care routine accordingly. Consistency and patience are key to achieving healthy, glowing skin. If you have any concerns or specific skincare goals, keep reading let's see if we can tackle them. Severe issues consult with a licensed dermatologist for personalized advice and recommendations.

NOW HERE COMES THE FRUSTRATIONS WITH SOME SOLUTIONS:

- **Frustration**: Excess oiliness.
- **Solution**: Use oil-free, non-comedogenic products to control shine and prevent breakouts.(ie: Slipping makeup. makeup looks great on oily skin right after application, however no matter how much you spend on your makeup it will disappear after a short period of time)

- **Frustration**: Dry, flaky skin.

- **Solution**: Hydrate with rich, emollient moisturizers and incorporate hydrating serums into your routine.(ie: cakey makeup. If the skin is dehydrated, flaky, textured, or not in its best shape. this will result in how make-up sits on the skin)

- **Frustration**: Breakouts and acne which is not age specific.
- **Solution**: Treat acne with gentle yet effective ingredients like salicylic acid and benzoyl peroxide, and avoid harsh scrubbing or picking which leads to scarring, not that we cant help there too but prevention is better than cure

- **Frustration**: Hyperpigmentation and dark spots.
- **Solution**: Use brightening ingredients like vitamin C and niacin-amide to fade discoloration and even out skin tone.

- **Frustration**: Sensitive skin reactions.
- **Solution**: Opt for fragrance-free, hypoallergenic products and patch-test new products before applying them to your entire face.

- **Frustration**: Keloids and scars.
- **Solution**: Consult with a dermatologist for treatment options, which may include corticosteroid injections or silicone gel sheets.

- **Frustration**: Ashy, dull skin.

- **Solution:** Keep your skin moisturized with hydrating creams and oils, and exfoliate regularly to remove dead skin cells

- **Frustration**: Uneven skin texture.
- **Solution**: Incorporate chemical exfoliants like alpha hydroxy acids (AHAs) or beta hydroxy acids (BHAs) to smooth rough patches and refine skin texture.

- **Frustration**: Lack of elasticity.
- **Solution**: Use collagen-boosting. ingredients like retinoids and peptides to improve skin firmness and resilience.

- **Frustration**: Sun damage and photoaging.
- **Solution**: Protect your skin from UV rays with broad-spectrum sunscreen and wear protective clothing, hats, and sunglasses when outdoors.

Bet you didn't know:

🥴 Did you know that honey is a natural humectant that locks in moisture and soothes dry skin? Incorporate honey-based masks into your routine for a hydrating treat.

🤔Green tea isn't just for sipping - it's also packed with antioxidants that can help protect your skin from environmental damage. Brew up a cup and use it as a toner for a refreshing boost. Simply steep green teabag in hot water, allow it to cool, then apply it to your skin using a cotton pad. The antioxidants in green tea will help to soothe inflammation, reduce redness and provide a gentle, revitalizing effect for your skin.

😳Did you know that shea butter is a skincare powerhouse? This natural emollient is rich in vitamins and fatty acids, making it perfect for moisturizing dry skin, soothing irritation, and promoting elasticity.

WE'RE NOT JUST SELLING PRODUCTS, WE'RE BUILDING A TRIBE WHILE EDUCATING

At pretti please beauty co., we understand the unique challenges faced by individuals with different skin types and different skin complexions, when it comes to skincare. That's why our products are specially formulated to address these concerns and help you achieve your skin goals with confidence.

- For those struggling with excess oiliness, our oil-balancing cleansers and lightweight moisturizers are designed to keep shine at bay without stripping the skin of essential moisture.
- If dry, flaky skin is your frustration, our hydrating formulas work to replenish moisture and restore skin's natural barrier, leaving you with a smooth, supple complexion.
- Combat breakouts and acne with our targeted treatments containing ingredients like salicylic acid and benzoyl peroxide, which help to clear blemishes and prevent future breakouts without irritating sensitive skin.
- Protect your skin from sunburn and sun damage

with our broad-spectrum sunscreens, formulated to shield your skin from harmful uv rays while providing lightweight, non-greasy protection.

- Soothe redness and irritation with our gentle, fragrance-free products, enriched with calming ingredients like aloe vera and chamomile to reduce inflammation and promote a more even skin tone.
- Address fine lines and wrinkles with our anti-aging serums and creams, packed with retinoids and antioxidants to stimulate collagen production and diminish signs of aging for a more youthful appearance.
- Revitalize dull, lackluster skin with our exfoliating scrubs and brightening treatments, which work to remove dead skin cells and reveal a brighter, more radiant complexion.
- Minimized sensitivity and irritation with our hypoallergenic formulations, carefully crafted to be gentle yet effective for even the most delicate skin types.
- Fade uneven skin tone and dark spots with our brightening products containing potent ingredients like vitamin C and NIACIN-AMIDE, which help to fade discoloration and promote a more uniform complexion.
- Refine pores and texture with our pore-minimizing serums and masks, formulated to smooth skin's surface and reduce the appearance of enlarged pores for a refined, flawless finish.
- With Pretti please beauty co skincare, you can trust that our products are backed by science and formulated with your skin's needs in mind. Say

goodbye to frustration and hello to radiant, healthy skin with our comprehensive range of skincare solutions. Let us be your partner on the journey to your best skin ever

At pretti please beauty co. we're dedicated to providing high-quality skincare solutions tailored to the unique needs of individuals. Fair skinned to richly Melanated and all the amazing colors In-between. Our products are formulated with carefully selected ingredients to address common skin concerns while promoting radiance, clarity, and vitality. Trust in our expertise and let us guide you on your journey to healthy, beautiful skin.

Pretti, Prepare to embark on a journey with the rest of your tribe and experience self-discovery and empowerment as you unlock the secrets to luminously, healthy skin with pretti please beauty co. Let us be your trusted partner on the path to beauty and confidence.

3 YOUR DAILY SKINCARE ROUTINE: A JOURNEY TO RADIANT SKIN

Welcome to your daily skincare sanctuary, where self-care meets science to unlock your skin's full potential. In this chapter, we'll guide you through the essential steps of a skincare routine tailored to your unique needs. Whether you're a skincare aficionado or a newbie to the beauty world, get ready to embark on a journey to Gorgeous, radiant, healthy skin!

Step-by-step skincare routine for all skin types:

1. Cleansing:

Start your day by gently cleansing your skin to remove impurities and prepare it for the day ahead. Choose a cleanser suited to your skin type—foaming for oily skin, cream for dry skin, or gel for combination skin.

2. Toning:

After cleansing, apply a toner to rebalance your skin's pH levels and refine pores. Look for toners with hydrating ingredients like hyaluronic acid or soothing botanical extracts.

3. Treatment:

Address specific skin concerns with targeted treatments, such as serums or spot treatments. Whether you're battling acne, hyperpigmentation, or fine lines, choose products formulated with active ingredients to deliver visible results.

4. Moisturizing:

Hydrate and nourish your skin with a moisturizer suitable for your skin type. Opt for lightweight, oil-free formulas for oily skin, or richer creams for dry skin. Don't forget to apply moisturizer to your neck and décolletage too!

5. Sun Protection:

Finish off your morning routine with broad-spectrum sunscreen to protect your skin from UV damage and premature aging. Choose a sunscreen with SPF 30 or higher and reapply throughout the day, especially if you'll be spending time outdoors.

6. Nighttime Renewal:

In the evening, repeat the cleansing and toning steps to remove makeup and impurities from the day. Follow up with any treatment products, allowing them to penetrate deeply into your skin while you sleep.

7. Overnight Hydration:

Seal in moisture with a nourishing night cream or sleeping mask to replenish your skin's hydration levels overnight. Wake up to plump, glowing skin ready to face the day ahead.

Skincare routine for the busy bee, because yeah sometimes life be lifing and you just don't have time:
(Don't worry, we got you covered with a simplified skincare routine that still packs a punch!)

1. Cleanse:

Streamline your morning routine with a multitasking cleanser that doubles as a toner. Look for gentle, all-in-one formulas that cleanse, tone, and refresh your skin in one step.

2. Treatment:

Treatment: Cut down on steps by using a multipurpose treatment product that addresses multiple concerns at once. Choose a serum or moisturizer with potent ingredients like vitamin C or hyaluronic acid to hydrate, brighten, and protect your skin in one go.

3. Protect:

Don't skip the sunscreen! Opt for a lightweight, tinted moisturizer with SPF to streamline your morning routine while still protecting your skin from UV damage.

4. Nighttime Refresh:

Keep your evening routine simple with a gentle cleanser followed by a hydrating night cream or sleeping mask. Let your skin soak up the nourishing ingredients overnight for a refreshed complexion come morning.

Trust in Pretti Please Beauty:

At pretti please beauty, we know that every moment counts when it comes to self-care and life in general that's why our products are thoughtfully formulated to deliver visible results without compromising on efficiency. Whether you have all the time in the world or just a few precious minutes, trust in our expertise to guide you on your journey to radiant, healthy skin.

Prepare to elevate your skincare routine with pretti please

beauty co, where science meets self-care to unlock your skin's full potential. Let's embark on this transformative journey together!

We're so glad you're here!!

4 THE POWER OF CLEANSING: CLEARING AWAY IMPURITIES

Welcome to the gateway to gorgeous skin—cleansing! In this chapter, we'll delve into the transformative power of cleansing and how it sets the stage for a skincare routine that leaves you glowing from within. Get ready to embark on a journey to discover the importance of cleansing, how to choose the perfect cleanser for your skin type, and how to incorporate self-care into your cleansing ritual.

The importance of cleansing:

Cleansing isn't just about removing makeup and dirt—it's about creating a clean canvas for your skincare products to work their magic. Throughout the day, our skin is exposed to pollutants, bacteria, and environmental toxins that can clog pores and lead to breakouts, dullness, and premature aging. Cleansing helps to remove these impurities, allowing your skin to breathe and absorb the nourishing ingredients in your skincare routine more effectively.

Choosing the Right Cleanser:

With so many cleansers on the market, finding the perfect match for your skin can feel like searching for a needle in a haystack. But fear not! We're here to guide you through the process and help you find the cleanser of your dreams.

1.Know Your Skin Type:

The first step in choosing a cleanser is understanding your skin type. Are you oily, dry, combination, or sensitive? Knowing your skin type will help you narrow down your options and find a cleanser that meets your skin's specific needs. All of our products have full ingredients in the DESCRIPTIONs.

2. Consider Your Concerns:

In addition to your skin type, consider any specific concerns you'd like to address, such as acne, aging, or hyperpigmentation. Look at our products formulated with ingredients that target these concerns, such as salicylic acid for acne-prone skin or hyaluronic acid for hydration.

3. Read the descriptions listed on our product pages and labels:

Pay attention to the ingredients list and avoid harsh chemicals and fragrances that can irritate sensitive skin. Look for gentle, non-comedogenic products that won't strip your skin of its natural oils.

4. Test it Out:

Test it Out: When trying a new cleanser, patch-test it on a small area of your skin before applying it to your entire face. This will help you determine if the cleanser is suitable for your skin and won't cause any adverse reactions.

Incorporating Self-Care into Your Cleansing Ritual: Let's pour into you:

• **Mindful moments:** take a few deep breaths and center yourself before beginning your cleansing ritual. Use this time to set intentions for your skincare routine and cultivate a sense of mindfulness and self-awareness.

• **Gentle massage:** as you cleanse your skin, take the opportunity to give yourself a gentle facial massage. Use circular motions to stimulate circulation, promote lymphatic drainage, and release tension in your facial muscles.

• **Sensory experience:** engage your senses by choosing a cleanser with a soothing scent or luxurious texture. Let the calming aroma and silky texture enhance your cleansing experience and transport you to a state of relaxation.

Fun Facts About Cleansing:

Did you know that the ancient Egyptians were among the first to use cleansing agents for skincare? They used a combination of oils and natural ingredients to cleanse and exfoliate their skin, paving the way for modern skincare rituals.

Cleansing isn't just for your face! Don't forget to cleanse your neck, chest, and back, as these areas are also prone to buildup of dirt and oil.

Double cleansing is a game-changer for removing makeup and sunscreen. Start with an oil-based cleanser to dissolve makeup and follow up with a water-based cleanser to remove any remaining impurities.

At Pretti Please Beauty, we believe in the power of cleansing to transform your skin and unleash your inner radiance. Our cleansers are thoughtfully formulated with gentle yet effective ingredients to cleanse, purify, and nourish your skin without stripping its natural moisture barrier. Trust in our expertise and let us guide you on your skin care journey

Prepare to elevate your cleansing ritual with pretti please beauty. Where science meets self-care to unlock your skin's full potential. Let's embark on this transformative journey together!

5 LET'S GET INTO NOURISHING YOUR SKIN: INGREDIENTS TO LOOK FOR

Now we enter the world of skincare alchemy, where potent ingredients come together to nourish and protect your skin. In this chapter, we'll delve into the fascinating realm of skincare ingredients, from antioxidants to hyaluronic acid, and uncover their transformative benefits for your skin. Get ready to discover the key ingredients to look for in your skincare products and how they can elevate your skincare routine to new heights of radiance and vitality.

The Power of Skincare Ingredients:

Skincare ingredients are the building blocks of a healthy, glowing complexion. From hydrating humectants to protective antioxidants, each ingredient plays a crucial role in nourishing and enhancing the health of your skin. By understanding the benefits of these ingredients, you can make informed choices about the products you use and achieve your skincare goals with confidence.

Key Ingredients to Look For:

1. Hyaluronic acid: a powerhouse hydrator, hyaluronic acid attracts moisture to the skin and helps to plump and firm the complexion. Look for products containing hyaluronic acid to replenish moisture and maintain a healthy skin barrier.

2. Vitamin C: a potent antioxidant, vitamin c helps to brighten the skin, fade dark spots, and protect against environmental damage. Incorporate vitamin c serums or moisturizers into your routine to promote a more even, radiant complexion.

3. Retinoids: derived from vitamin a, retinoids are powerhouse ingredients for anti-aging and acne treatment. They stimulate collagen production, reduce the appearance of fine lines and wrinkles, and help to unclog pores for a clearer, smoother complexion.

4. Niacin-amide: also known as vitamin b3, niacin-amide is a versatile ingredient that helps to improve skin texture, minimize pores, and reduce redness and inflammation. It's suitable for all skin types and can be found in serums, moisturizers, and toners.

5. Peptides: peptides are amino acid chains that help to stimulate collagen production and improve skin elasticity. Incorporate peptide-rich products into your routine to support skin renewal and maintain a youthful, plump complexion.

6. Antioxidants: antioxidants like green tea extract, resveratrol, and vitamin E help to protect the skin from oxidative stress and environmental damage caused by free radicals. Look for products containing antioxidants to shield your skin from premature aging and maintain its youthful vitality.

7. Glycolic acid: a type of alpha hydroxy acid (aha), glycolic acid gently exfoliates the skin, removing dead cells and promoting cell turnover. It helps to improve skin texture, reduce the appearance of fine lines and wrinkles, and enhance the effectiveness of other skincare ingredients.

8. Ceramides: essential lipids found in the skin's natural barrier, ceramides help to lock in moisture and protect against environmental aggressors. Look for ceramide-rich products to strengthen your skin's barrier function and prevent moisture loss.

9. Squalene: a lightweight moisturizing agent derived from olives, squalene helps to hydrate and nourish the skin without clogging pores. It's suitable for all skin types and can be found in serums, moisturizers, and facial oils.

10. Aloe vera: known for its soothing and hydrating properties, aloe vera is a natural healer for irritated or inflamed skin. Incorporate products containing aloe vera to calm redness, reduce inflammation, and promote overall skin health.

There are significantly more ingredients that we will follow up with in later releases:

Incorporating ingredients into your skincare routine:

- **Layering:** Experiment with layering different skincare ingredients to maximize their benefits. Start with lightweight serums containing water-soluble ingredients like vitamin C or niacinamide, followed by heavier creams or oils containing lipid-soluble ingredients like retinoids or ceramides.

- **Consistency:** Consistency is key when it comes to seeing results from skincare ingredients. Stick to your routine and give your skin time to adjust to new products, usually around 4-6 weeks, before expecting to see noticeable improvements.

- **Patch Testing:** Before incorporating new ingredients into your routine, it's important to patch-test them on a small area of your skin to check for any adverse reactions. Apply a small amount of product to your inner arm or behind your ear and wait 24-48 hours to see if any irritation occurs.

At Pretti Please Beauty Co, we believe in the power of science-backed ingredients to nourish and transform your skin. Our products are formulated with carefully selected ingredients to deliver visible results without compromising on safety or efficacy. we don't gamble with your skin we rely on facts, science and cruelty free testing with all the ingredients we incorporate into our products.

6 HYDRATION: KEEPING YOUR SKIN SUPPLE AND MOISTURIZED

Whew, the oasis of hydration, where moisture meets magic to unveil your skin's natural beauty. here we'll delve into the essential role of hydration in maintaining youthful, supple skin for all skin types and explore how to incorporate hydrating products into your skincare routine. Get ready to dive deep into the world of moisture and discover the secrets to a dewy complexion that glows from within.

The importance of hydration:

Hydration is the cornerstone of healthy, radiant skin. Just like our bodies need water to function optimally, our skin relies on hydration to maintain its moisture balance, elasticity, and overall health. When our skin is properly hydrated, it looks plump, smooth, and youthful, while dehydration can lead to dullness, dryness, and premature aging

Quiz: how hydrated is your skin?

Take this quick quiz to assess the hydration level of your skin:

1. How does your skin feel after cleansing?

• A) Tight and dry

• B) Soft and comfortable

• C) Oily or greasy

2. Do you experience flakiness or rough texture?

• A) Yes, frequently

• B) Occasionally

• C) Rarely

3. How often do you experience dry patches or irritation?

• A) Often

• B) Sometimes

• C) Rarely or never

4. How does your skin appear throughout the day?

• A) Dull and lackluster

• B) Fresh and radiant

• C) Shiny or oily

5. Do you notice fine lines or wrinkles?

• A) Yes, they're prominent

• B) Yes, but they're minimal

• C) No, my skin is smooth

RESULTS:

• **Mostly A's:** your skin may be dehydrated and in need of extra moisture.

• **Mostly B's:** your skin is adequately hydrated, but could benefit from additional hydration.

• **Mostly C's:** your skin is well-hydrated and balanced.

Don't fret pretti, 93% of our customers started with mostly A's before using our products

Incorporating Hydration into Your Skincare Routine:

1. Choose the right moisturizer: look for moisturizers with hydrating ingredients like hyaluronic acid, glycerin, and ceramides. These ingredients help to attract and lock in moisture, keeping your skin plump and supple throughout the day. All of pretti please beauty products have hydrating formulas built in.

2. Layer: hydrating products: experiment with layering

hydrating serums, essences, and facial oils to boost moisture levels and address specific concerns like dryness or dehydration. Start with lighter textures and build up to richer formulas as needed.

3. Don't forget sunscreen: sunscreen is essential for protecting your skin from uv damage, which can lead to dehydration and premature aging. Choose a moisturizer with built-in SPF or layer sunscreen over your moisturizer for added protection. All of pretti please beauty moisturizing products have sunscreen protection

4. Hydrate from within: remember to drink plenty of water throughout the day to hydrate your skin from the inside out. Aim for at least eight glasses of water daily, and incorporate hydrating foods like fruits and vegetables into your diet for an extra moisture boost.

The pinch test:

A simple way to assess your skin's hydration level is by performing the pinch test. Pinch a small area of skin on the back of your hand and hold for a few seconds, then release. If your skin bounces back quickly, it's well-hydrated. If it takes longer to bounce back or remains "tented," it may be dehydrated and in need of moisture.

Hydration and Self-Care:

Incorporating hydration into your skincare routine is not only essential for maintaining healthy skin but also an act of self-care. Taking the time to nourish your skin with hydrating products is a form of self-love, allowing you to pamper yourself and prioritize your well-being. So, embrace the ritual of hydration as a moment of indulgence and relaxation, and let it rejuvenate not only your skin but also your soul.

Pretti known fact:

Did you know that up to 60% of the human adult body is water? That's why staying hydrated is crucial for overall health and well-being, including the health of your skin!

Trust us, we got you:

We at pretti please beauty co. Understand the importance of hydration for healthy, glowing skin. That's why our products are formulated with hydrating ingredients to nourish and replenish your skin's moisture barrier, leaving it soft, smooth, and supple.

We were where you are once too and know the importance. Trust in our expertise and let us guide you on your journey to dewy, hydrated skin.

7 PROTECTING YOUR BEAUTIFUL SKIN: SUNSCREEN AND BEYOND

Before we start lets get this out the way so everyone reads this chapter.

People of darker pigmentations do not need sunscreen!

Myth: studies have shown if an individual goes outdoors and the sun touches their skin they need sunscreen, regardless of skin color.

Sun protection is paramount for preventing premature aging and protecting against harmful uv rays. Learn about the importance of sunscreen and other ways to shield your skin from environmental damage.

Sunscreen is the fortress of protection, where your skin's shield against the elements is fortified. In this chapter, we'll explore the critical role of sun protection in preventing premature aging and safeguarding against harmful uv rays. Get ready to dive into the importance of sunscreen and discover additional ways to shield your skin from environmental damage, all while prioritizing self-care and incorporating insightful studies.

The importance of sun protection:

Sun protection isn't just about preventing sunburn—it's about defending your skin against long-term damage that can lead to wrinkles, sun spots, and even skin cancer. Uv rays from the sun can penetrate the skin's layers, causing DNA damage and accelerating the aging process. By incorporating sun protection into your daily routine, you can shield your skin from harm and maintain a youthful, healthy complexion for years to come.

Self-care and sun protection:

Caring for your skin goes hand in hand with caring for yourself. Sun protection isn't just a skincare step—it's an act of self-care that shows your skin the love and attention it deserves. By prioritizing sun protection, you're not only safeguarding your skin's health but also nurturing your overall well-being. So, embrace the ritual of sunscreen application as a moment of mindfulness and self-preservation, and let it become a cornerstone of your daily self-care routine.

The sunscreen study:

A recent study published in the journal of the American academy of dermatology found that regular sunscreen use can significantly reduce the risk of skin aging caused by sun exposure. Participants who applied sunscreen daily showed fewer signs of aging, including wrinkles, sagging, and sun spots, compared to those who didn't use sunscreen consistently. This highlights the importance of incorporating sunscreen into your skincare regimen to protect against premature aging and maintain a youthful complexion.

Beyond sunscreen: additional ways to protect your skin:

1. Seek shade: whenever possible, seek shade during peak sun hours (10 a.m. To 4 p.m.) To reduce your overall sun exposure and minimize the risk of sunburn and skin damage.

2. Wear protective clothing: invest in clothing with UPF (ultraviolet protection factor) to provide an additional layer of defense against uv rays. Opt for long sleeves, wide-brimmed hats, and sunglasses to shield your skin and eyes from the sun's harmful rays.

3. Stay hydrated: hydrated skin is more resilient to sun damage, so be sure to drink plenty of water throughout the day to keep your skin hydrated from the inside out.

4. Antioxidant-rich skincare: incorporate skincare products containing antioxidants like vitamin c and e to help neutralize free radicals and protect against oxidative stress caused by uv exposure.

Please, please, please, Pretti Please! Protect your skin

Understand the importance of sun protection for maintaining healthy, glowing skin. That's why our products are formulated with broad-spectrum SPF and antioxidant-rich ingredients to provide comprehensive protection against environmental damage. Trust in our expertise and let us guide you on your journey to sun-safe, glowing, healthy skin.

8 SPECIAL TREATMENTS: MASKS, SERUMS, AND TREATMENTS

Indulge in the luxurious world of special skincare treatments that go beyond your daily routine. From decadent scrubs and butters to potent serums and targeted treatments, discover how these skincare treasures can elevate your regimen to new heights of indulgence and efficacy.

What Are Special Treatments?

Special treatments encompass a wide range of skincare products designed to address specific concerns or provide an extra boost of nourishment and hydration to your skin. From masks that deeply cleanse and hydrate to serums packed with potent active ingredients, these products offer targeted solutions to enhance the health and appearance of your skin.

Why Incorporate Special Treatments?

While your daily skincare routine lays the foundation for healthy skin, special treatments offer additional benefits and targeted solutions to address specific concerns. Whether you're looking to brighten, hydrate, or firm your skin, incorporating special treatments into your regimen can help you achieve your skincare goals more effectively and efficiently.

Where to Buy Special Treatments:

When it comes to purchasing special treatments for your skincare routine, it's essential to choose products from reputable brands that prioritize quality and efficacy. Look no further than Pretti Please Beauty Co. for a curated selection of masks, serums, lotions, butters and treatments formulated with premium ingredients to deliver visible results. Visit our website or explore our product range at select retailers to discover the perfect additions to your skincare arsenal.

Self-Care and Special Treatments:

Incorporating special treatments into your skincare routine isn't just about pampering your skin—it's also an act of self-care that nurtures your overall well-being. Taking the time to treat yourself to a luxurious mask or potent serum allows you to indulge in moments of relaxation and rejuvenation, fostering a deeper connection with yourself and your skin. So, embrace the ritual of special treatments as a form of self-love and self-preservation, and let them become a cherished part of your self-care routine.

Explore the World of Special Treatments with Pretti Please Beauty:

We believe in the transformative power of special treatments to elevate your skincare routine and unleash your skin's full potential. From our luxurious masks infused with nourishing botanicals to our potent serums enriched with active ingredients, each product is meticulously formulated to deliver visible results and a luxurious sensory experience.

9 MINDFUL BEAUTY: THE CONNECTION BETWEEN MENTAL HEALTH AND SKINCARE

Mindful beauty!!! Huh? Mindful beauty is where the profound connection between mental health and skincare unfolds.here we're ready to delve into the intricate relationship between our inner well-being and outer radiance, exploring how mindfulness techniques can enhance your beauty routine and nurture both your skin and soul.

The mind-body connection:

The mind-body connection is a fundamental principle that underscores the profound interplay between our mental and physical health. When it comes to skincare, our emotional well-being can have a significant impact on the health and appearance of our skin. Stress, anxiety, and negative emotions can manifest on the skin in various ways, from breakouts and inflammation to dullness and premature aging. By cultivating a positive mindset and practicing mindfulness, we can support our skin's health and enhance its natural beauty from within.

Why mental health matters for skincare:

Our skin is not just a superficial barrier—it's a reflection of our inner state of health and well-being. Stress and other emotional factors can disrupt the delicate balance of our skin, leading to a range of concerns such as acne, eczema, and premature aging. By prioritizing mental health and incorporating mindfulness techniques into our daily routine, we can reduce stress levels, promote relaxation, and support our skin's natural healing processes, resulting in a clearer, more radiant complexion.

Mindfulness techniques for beauty:

1. Meditation: dedicate a few minutes each day to quieting the mind and centering yourself through meditation. Focus on your breath, observe your thoughts without judgment, and cultivate a sense of inner calm and serenity. This practice not only reduces stress but also promotes a positive mindset and enhances your overall well-being, which is reflected in the health of your skin.

2. Gratitude practice: cultivate gratitude by reflecting on the things you're thankful for each day. Whether it's the warmth of the sun on your skin or the gentle touch of a skincare product, expressing gratitude can shift your perspective and elevate your mood, fostering a sense of contentment and inner peace. This positive outlook not only enhances your mental health but also radiates through your skin, giving it a healthy, luminous glow.

3. Breathing exercises: incorporate deep breathing exercises into your skincare routine to promote relaxation and reduce stress levels. Take slow, deep breaths in through your nose, filling your lungs with air, then exhale slowly through your mouth, releasing tension and calming your mind. This simple practice can help alleviate anxiety and promote a sense of tranquility, allowing your skin to thrive in a stress-free environment.

4. Mindful skincare rituals: transform your skincare

routine into a mindful ritual by savoring each step and fully engaging your senses. Pay attention to the textures, scents, and sensations of your skincare products as you apply them, allowing yourself to be fully present in the moment. This mindful approach not only enhances the efficacy of your skincare products but also deepens your connection with yourself and your skin.

Where and how to find mindful beauty products:

When it comes to incorporating self care and mindfulness into your beauty routine, choose products that nourish both your skin and soul. Pretti please beauty products offer a selection of skincare products infused with mindfulness and intention. Our products are meticulously formulated with premium ingredients to nourish your skin from the inside out, while our commitment to mindfulness ensures that each product is a sensorial experience that nurtures your overall well-being. Visit our website and explore our range of products to discover the perfect additions to your mindful beauty routine. You will be able to indulge in the luxury tranquil essence of the pretti please beauty collection, where every product is a journey to serenity. Elevate your senses with our warm, spa-inspired aromas, hand crafted and formulated to evoke moments of meditation, relaxation, inspiration, pure joy and self care. Discover the power of scent to uplift your spirit and embrace the beauty of inner peace.

10 BEAUTY FROM WITHIN: NUTRITION FOR RADIANT SKIN

Healthy skin starts from within. Learn about the role of nutrition in skincare and discover foods that promote a radiant complexion.

foods you eat play a vital role in achieving a radiant complexion. In this chapter, we'll explore the fascinating link between nutrition and skincare, uncovering the power of food to promote healthy, glowing skin. Get ready to embark on a delicious adventure that nourishes your skin from the inside out!

The Role of Nutrition in Skincare:

Healthy skin is a reflection of what you put into your body. Just as a balanced diet supports overall health, it also plays a crucial role in maintaining the health and appearance of your skin. Nutrient-rich foods provide essential vitamins, minerals, and antioxidants that support skin health, combatting inflammation, and promoting collagen production for a radiant complexion.

Fun Fact:

Did you know that dark chocolate contains flavonoids, antioxidants that can help protect your skin from sun damage and improve skin texture? Indulging in a square of dark chocolate can be a delicious way to support your skin's health and glow!

Quiz time: Discover Your Skin-Boosting Foods:

Take this interactive quiz to uncover which skin-boosting foods are best suited to your skincare needs:

1. Which of the following foods is rich in vitamin c, an antioxidant that helps brighten the skin and promote collagen production?

• A) Oranges

• B) Avocado

• C) Spinach

2. Which omega-3 fatty acid-rich food can help reduce inflammation and support skin hydration?

• A) Salmon

• B) Quinoa

• C) Broccoli

3. Which vitamin e-rich food helps protect the skin from oxidative damage and supports healthy cell turnover?

• A) Almonds

• B) Chicken breast

• C) White rice

4. Which antioxidant-rich food can help fight free radical

damage and promote a youthful complexion?

• A) Blueberries

• B) Beef

• C) Potatoes

Results:

• **Mostly A's:** your skin may benefit from incorporating more fruits like oranges and berries into your diet.

• **Mostly B's:** focus on adding omega-3 rich foods like salmon and nuts to support skin hydration and reduce inflammation.

• **Mostly C's:** increase your intake of vitamin e-rich foods like almonds and leafy greens to protect your skin from oxidative damage and promote healthy cell turnover.

Where to Find Skin-Boosting Foods:

When it comes to nourishing your skin from within, look no further than your local grocery store or farmer's market for an abundance of skin-boosting foods. Incorporate a variety of fruits, vegetables, lean proteins, and healthy fats into your diet to support your skin's health and radiance.

11 STRESS MANAGEMENT: TECHNIQUES FOR INNER PEACE AND BALANCE

Indulge in the Luxury Tranquil Essence of The Pretti Please Beauty Collection, where every product is a journey to serenity. Elevate your senses with our warm, spa-inspired aromas, hand crafted and formulated to evoke moments of meditation, relaxation, inspiration, pure joy and self care. Discover the power of scent to uplift your spirit and embrace the beauty of inner peace.

Welcome to the sanctuary of serenity, where stress melts away, and inner peace prevails. In this chapter, we'll embark on a journey to explore effective stress management techniques to uplift your spirit, soothe your soul, and rejuvenate your skin. Get ready to lighten the load and discover the joy of finding balance amidst life's chaos.

The Link Between Stress and Skin:

Stress isn't just a mental burden—it can also wreak havoc on your skin. When we're stressed, our bodies release cortisol, a hormone that can lead to inflammation, breakouts, and accelerated aging. By managing stress effectively, we can not only improve our mental well-being but also protect the health and beauty of our skin.

Fun Fact: Did you know that laughter can actually benefit your skin? When you laugh, your body releases endorphins, neurotransmitters that promote feelings of happiness and relaxation. These endorphins can help reduce stress levels, leading to a more radiant complexion and a brighter outlook on life!

Stress-Relieving Strategy: Laughter Therapy

Laughter truly is the best medicine, and incorporating laughter therapy into your daily routine can be a powerful tool for stress management. Whether it's watching a funny movie, sharing jokes with friends, or simply indulging in a hearty chuckle, laughter has the power to uplift your spirits and melt away stress.

You ever notice people with glowing skin are always smiling and look happy?

Fun Stress-Relieving Activities:

1. Watch funny movies or show: grab the remote, turn on your favorite streaming network and go to comedy. Look for Steve Harvey or Kevin Hart and prepare for the laughter to begin. Turn on a Tyler Perry movie such as "Madea" and let loose. Hours of spontaneous laughter, in the comfort of your own home. Laughing is a great way to release tension, boost your mood, and get your heart pumping for a natural endorphin rush.

2. Pamper yourself: treat yourself to a pampering session with indulgent skincare products and luxurious bath essentials. Create a spa-like atmosphere with candles, soothing music, and your favorite scents to melt away stress and rejuvenate your mind, body, and soul.

3. Creative outlet: engage in a creative activity that brings you joy, whether it's painting, writing, or crafting. Channeling your creativity can help you express yourself, process emotions, and find solace amidst the chaos of daily life.

4. Nature walk: take a leisurely stroll and immerse yourself in the beauty of the outdoors. It doesn't matter if your in an urban area or the suburbs you can always connect with nature. Studies have shown that mindfulness and connecting with nature reduces stress levels and promote a sense of calm and well-being, making it the perfect antidote to a hectic day.

12 THE IMPORTANCE OF SLEEP: BEAUTY REST FOR GLOWING SKIN

The realm of beauty rest, where quality sleep is the secret to a radiant complexion. In this chapter, we'll explore the vital role of sleep in skin repair and rejuvenation and uncover simple strategies to optimize your sleep hygiene for healthy, glowing skin.

The Link Between Sleep and Skin Health:

Quality sleep is not just a luxury—it's a necessity for maintaining healthy, beautiful skin. During sleep, your body undergoes crucial repair processes, including the production of collagen and cell turnover, which are essential for maintaining skin elasticity and combating signs of aging. By prioritizing sleep, you can support your skin's natural regeneration process and wake up to a brighter, more refreshed complexion.

Get More Sleep Strategy:

1. Establish a bedtime routine: create a calming bedtime routine to signal to your body that it's time to wind down and prepare for sleep. This could include activities such as reading, gentle stretching, or practicing relaxation techniques like deep breathing or meditation.

2. Limit screen time: minimize exposure to screens, such as smartphones, tablets, and computers, at least an hour before bedtime. The blue light emitted by electronic devices can disrupt your body's natural sleep-wake cycle and make it harder to fall asleep.

3. Create a restful environment: make your bedroom a sanctuary for sleep by keeping it cool, dark, and quiet. Invest in a comfortable mattress and pillows and consider using blackout curtains or a white noise machine to create an optimal sleeping environment.

4. Avoid stimulants: limit your intake of caffeine, nicotine, and alcohol, especially in the hours leading up to bedtime. These substances can interfere with your ability to fall asleep and disrupt the quality of your sleep throughout the night.

Quiz: How Much Sleep Are You Getting?

Take this quick quiz to assess your sleep habits and discover if you're getting enough rest:

1. What time do you typically go to bed?

• A) Before 10 p.m.

• B) Between 10 p.m. and midnight

• C) After'''' midnight

2. How many hours of sleep do you get on weeknights?

• A) 7-9 hours

• B) 6-7 hours

• C) Less than 6 hours

3. Do you feel well-rested and refreshed when you wake

up in the morning?

- A) Yes, most of the time

- B) Occasionally

- C) Rarely or never

Results:

- **Mostly A's:** you're likely getting sufficient sleep and prioritizing your rest. Keep up the good work!

- **Mostly B's:** you may be getting an adequate amount of sleep, but there's room for improvement. Focus on optimizing your sleep hygiene to ensure better quality rest.

- **Mostly C's:** you may be experiencing sleep deprivation, which can take a toll on your skin and overall health. Consider making changes to your sleep habits to prioritize rest and rejuvenation.

13 EXERCISE AND SKIN HEALTH: A HEALTHY BODY, A HEALTHY GLOW

The dynamic duo of exercise and skin health, where getting active not only benefits your body but also enhances your skin's natural radiance. In this chapter, we'll explore the symbiotic relationship between exercise and skin health, and uncover simple workouts to promote a healthy, glowing complexion.

The link between exercise and skin health:

Exercise isn't just about toning muscles and improving cardiovascular health—it also plays a vital role in maintaining radiant skin. When you exercise, your body increases blood flow, delivering oxygen and nutrients to your skin cells and carrying away waste products and toxins. This increased circulation promotes a healthy complexion, giving your skin a natural glow from within.

Get more exercise:

1. Find activities you enjoy: incorporate activities that you genuinely enjoy into your exercise routine, whether it's dancing, hiking, swimming, or practicing yoga. Choosing activities that bring you joy makes it easier to stay consistent and maintain a healthy lifestyle.

2. Make movement a habit: incorporate movement into your daily routine by taking the stairs instead of the elevator, walking or biking to nearby destinations, or scheduling regular breaks to stretch and move throughout the day. Every little bit of movement counts towards your overall health and well-being.

3. Mix it up: keep your exercise routine interesting and engaging by trying new activities and workouts regularly. This not only prevents boredom but also challenges different muscle groups and promotes overall fitness and flexibility.

4. Prioritize recovery: remember to prioritize rest and recovery to allow your body and skin to replenish and rejuvenate after exercise. Ensure you're getting enough sleep, staying hydrated, and nourishing your body with nutrient-rich foods to support your skin's health and vitality.

Quiz: How Active Are You?

Take this quick quiz to assess your activity level and discover if you're getting enough exercise:

1. How many days per week do you engage in moderate to vigorous physical activity (e.g., brisk walking, jogging, cycling)?

- A) 5-7 days

- B) 3-4 days

- C) 1-2 days

- D) Rarely or never

2. How do you feel after exercising?

- A) Energized and refreshed

- B) Slightly tired but satisfied

- C) Exhausted and drained

3. Do you incorporate strength training exercises into your routine?

- A) Yes, regularly

- B) Occasionally

- C) No, not at all

Results?

Mostly A's: congratulations! You're consistently active and prioritizing your health and well-being.

Mostly B's: you're making an effort to stay active, but there's room for improvement. Consider incorporating more movement into your daily routine to boost your overall fitness and skin health.

Mostly C's: You may not be getting enough exercise to support your skin's health and vitality. Look for opportunities to incorporate more physical activity into your daily life and reap the benefits of a healthy, glowing complexion.

In this chapter, we've explored the symbiotic relationship between exercise and skin health, and uncovered simple workouts to promote a healthy, glowing complexion.

Conclusion:

As you embark on your journey to better skin health through exercise, remember that consistency is key. Incorporating regular physical activity into your routine not only supports your overall well-being but also nourishes your skin from within. Whether you're breaking a sweat in the gym, taking a leisurely walk in nature, or practicing yoga in the comfort of your own home, each movement brings you one step closer to a healthier, more radiant complexion.

14 FINDING YOUR BALANCE: WORK, LIFE, AND SELF-CARE

Hey Pretti! Let's chat about finding that elusive thing called balance, shall we? Balancing work, life, and self-care might feel like juggling flaming torches sometimes, but trust me, it's essential for keeping that sparkle in your eye and that glow on your skin. So, grab a cup of tea, cozy up, and let's uncover some strategies for finding your equilibrium and putting self-care front and center in your daily routine.

Navigating the chaos:

Life can life. When life starts life-ing it becomes balance where? Between deadlines, family obligations, and just, you know, adulting in general, finding balance can feel like searching for a unicorn. But fear not! With a little bit of intention and a sprinkle of self-love, we can tame the chaos and create space for the things that truly matter.

Prioritizing self-care:

Repeat after me: self-care isn't selfish—it's essential. Carving out time for yourself isn't just a luxury; it's a necessity for maintaining your sanity and nurturing your well-being. Whether it's indulging in a skincare ritual, taking a bubble bath, or simply enjoying a moment of peace and quiet, make self-care a non-negotiable part of your daily routine.

The Power of Boundaries:

Setting boundaries isn't just about saying no—it's about saying yes to yourself. Learn to prioritize your needs and honor your limits, whether it's setting aside time for relaxation, saying no to extra commitments, or unplugging from technology when you need a break. Remember, you can't pour from an empty cup, so fill yours up first.

Embracing Imperfection:

Spoiler alert: nobody has it all together all the time, and that's perfectly okay. Embrace the messiness of life, celebrate your victories (big or small), and give yourself permission to be perfectly imperfect. After all, it's the bumps in the road that make the journey memorable, right?

Pretti take care of you:

Pretti Please Beauty Co, we believe that self-care isn't just a buzzword or a trend—it's a way of life and should be normalized. Our products are designed to nourish your skin and nurture your soul, providing a little slice of indulgence in your everyday routine. So, go ahead, treat yourself to a moment of pampering, because you deserve it, pretti.

As you navigate the balancing act of life, remember to prioritize yourself and indulge in a little self-care along the way. With a sprinkle of kindness and a dash of intention, you'll find your balance and glow from the inside out. Cheers to finding harmony and radiance in every moment! Remember you are part of a tribe of beautiful people!

15 SELF-CARE RITUALS: CREATING MOMENTS OF JOY AND RELAXATION

OK, Pretti! So, we've talked about finding balance in the chaos of life, right? Now, let's dive into the fun part—self-care rituals! Because let's be real, taking care of yourself isn't just about slathering on skincare products (although that's definitely part of it). It's about treating yourself with kindness, indulging in little moments of joy, and embracing relaxation like it's your job. So, grab your favorite cozy blanket and get ready to explore some self-care rituals that'll make your heart sing and your skin glow.

Mindful Moments:

Picture this: you're sitting in your favorite cozy corner, surrounded by flickering candles (which we have coming soon, innocent plug, lol) with soft music playing in the background. You take a deep breath and let go of all the stress and tension from the day. This, pretti, is the magic of mindfulness. Whether it's practicing meditation, journaling, manifesting or simply taking a few moments to breathe deeply, incorporating mindful moments into your day can work wonders for your well-being.

Indulgent Baths:

Ah, the glorious ritual of soaking in a warm bath—it's like a hug for your soul. Add a herbal tea bag soak from pretti please beauty co and maybe some bubbles, and let the warm water envelop you in its embrace. Bonus points if you bring along a good book or your favorite playlist for some extra relaxation. Trust me, a luxurious bath is the ultimate act of self-love.

Skincare Sanctuary:

Okay, okay, I know we said self-care isn't just about skincare, but hear me out: there's something truly magical about pampering your skin. Whether it's slathering on a hydrating face mask, giving yourself a soothing massage with a facial oil, or simply taking the time to cleanse away the day's impurities, your skin will thank you for the extra love and attention.

Connection and Community:

Self-care isn't just a solo endeavor—it's about connecting with others and building a community of support and love. Whether it's spending time with friends and family, joining a fitness class, or volunteering for a cause you care about, nurturing your relationships and fostering connections is an essential part of self-care.

Building a Supportive Community: Surrounding Yourself with Positivity:

Let's face it, life's too short to surround yourself with anything but good energy, am I right? So, grab a cup of tea and let's dive into why building a supportive community is not only great for your mental health but also for keeping that radiant glow on your skin.

The Importance of Positivity:

Okay, picture this: you're hanging out with your favorite people, laughing until your sides hurt, and feeling like you can take on the world. That, my friend, is the magic of positivity. Surrounding yourself with uplifting vibes and supportive individuals can do wonders for your mood, mindset, and yes, even your skin.

Nurturing Meaningful Connections:

Ever heard the saying, "your vibe attracts your tribe"? Well, it's true! Investing time and energy into nurturing meaningful connections with like-minded individuals can create a sense of belonging and support that's invaluable. Whether it's bonding over shared interests, offering a listening ear, or simply being there for each other through life's ups and downs, these connections nourish your soul and add a little extra sparkle to your life.

Creating a Safe Space:

Your community should be a safe haven—a place where you feel accepted, valued, and supported for who you are. Surround yourself with people who lift you up, inspire you to be your best self, and cheer you on every step of the way. Together, you'll create a space filled with love, laughter, and endless possibilities.

Spreading Kindness and Positivity:

Remember, positivity is contagious! By spreading kindness and positivity wherever you go, you not only uplift others but also cultivate a brighter, happier world for yourself. Whether it's offering a compliment, lending a helping hand, or simply sharing a smile with a stranger, every act of kindness contributes to the collective positivity of your community.

We at Pretti Please Beauty Co. believe in the power of positivity and community to uplift and inspire. That's why our products are more than just skincare—they're a reflection of our commitment to spreading love, joy, and happiness in the world. So, surround yourself with positivity, Pretti, and let your inner glow shine bright.

Self-care is a holistic experience that encompasses mind, body, and soul. That's why our products are designed to not only nourish your skin but also uplift your spirit and bring moments of joy and relaxation into your life. So, go ahead, indulge in a little self-care, my friend. You deserve it.

As you embrace the magic of self-care rituals, build your supportive community and surround yourself with POSITIVITY. remember that you are creating a space where you can thrive, grow and shine. Always remember to savor the moments of joy and relaxation that they bring. With a sprinkle of intention, a dash of indulgence, a little love, laughter, and a whole lot of positivity, you'll create a sanctuary of self-love and support that nourishes your soul and keeps your skin glowing from the inside out. Here's to finding bliss in every moment and building a life filled with love and light!

Welcome to the pretti tribe

16 EMBRACING IMPERFECTION: THE BEAUTY OF SELF-ACCEPTANCE

Hey there, pretti! Can you believe we're nearing the end of our journey together? But before we say goodbye, let's dive into one final topic that's close to my heart: the beauty of imperfection and the liberation of self-acceptance. Because let's be real, life's too short to strive for perfection when embracing our unique quirks and qualities is where the true magic lies. So, grab a cozy blanket and let's cozy up for a heart-to-heart about the beauty of imperfection and why learning to love ourselves exactly as we are is the ultimate act of self-care.

The Myth of Perfection:

Let's bust a little myth, shall we? Perfection? Yeah, it's overrated. In a world that's constantly bombarding us with images of flawless beauty and unattainable standards, it's easy to fall into the trap of chasing an ideal that doesn't even exist. But here's the thing: imperfection is what makes us human, and it's in those beautifully flawed moments that our true essence shines brightest.

Finding Beauty in Imperfection:

Have you ever looked in the mirror and noticed all the little things that make you uniquely you? The freckles sprinkled across your nose, the laugh lines that tell the story of a life well-lived, the quirks and quirks that make you unmistakably you? That, my friend, is the beauty of imperfection. It's in those perfectly imperfect moments that our true beauty shines through, radiating from the inside out.

The Liberation of Self-Acceptance:

Imagine a life where you wake up every morning, look in the mirror, and smile at the reflection staring back at you—not because you're flawless, but because you're perfectly imperfect and utterly beautiful in your own unique way. That, my friend, is the liberation of self-acceptance. It's the freedom to embrace every aspect of yourself, flaws and all, with love, kindness, and compassion.

True beauty lies in embracing our imperfections and celebrating our unique qualities. That's why our products are more than just skincare—they're a reminder to love yourself exactly as you are and to treat your skin with the kindness and care it deserves. So, as you continue on your journey of self-acceptance, know that we're here cheering you on every step of the way.

As we wrap up our time together, remember that imperfection is not something to be fixed or hidden—it's something to be celebrated and embraced. So, here's to embracing our quirks, loving ourselves fiercely, and radiating beauty from the inside out. Thank you for joining me on this journey, my friend. Until we meet again, may your heart be light, your spirit be bright, and your skin be positively radiant. Cheers to the beauty of imperfection and the joy of self-acceptance.

17 CONCLUSION: EMBRACING YOUR RADIANCE

Dear friend,

As we come to the end of our transformative skincare journey together, i want to express my deepest gratitude for sharing this adventure with me. Throughout our exploration of self-care, we've delved into the world of skincare rituals, positivity, and self-acceptance, forming a bond that transcends mere words on a page.

Your skincare journey is not just about achieving a flawless complexion—it's about embracing the journey of self-discovery, self-love, and self-acceptance. It's about nurturing your skin and soul with intention and kindness and allowing your inner radiance to shine brightly for the world to see.

At Pretti Please Beauty Co., we understand the profound impact that self-care can have on one's life and skin, and we're honored to be a part of your skincare journey. Our products are crafted with care and intention, designed to nourish your skin and elevate your self-care rituals to moments of pure indulgence and joy.

But our journey doesn't end here—it's only just beginning. As a cherished member of our skincare community, you're not just a customer—you're a part of our tribe, a beacon of light in a world that sometimes feels dim. So, as you continue on your skincare journey, know that we're here for you every step of the way, cheering you on, lifting you up, and celebrating your beauty, both inside and out.

Thank you, from the bottom of my heart, for entrusting us with your skincare journey. Together, let's continue to embrace our radiance, spread love and positivity, and shine brightly for all the world to see.

With love and gratitude,

Niccol A

Pretti Please Beauty Co.

ABOUT THE AUTHOR

The Founder: Niccol A.

The Brand: Pretti Please Beauty Co. (Pretti Please Beauty, Pretti Please Beauty Lounge, etc.)

The Book: Skincare Starts With Self-care (2024)

Skincare Starts With Self-Care is a firsthand account of a beauty professional whom has adapted to the many changes and trends in the beauty field for over a decade, surviving turbulent times economically and culturally. It reads like an letter to a friend or a sit down over tea for a fun day out.

Niccol A is a beauty professional, Estetrician and chemist with over two decades of experience working with skincare, hair care and facials. Niccol owns two beauty lounges that focus on skincare, teeth whitening, hair care, facials, full body treatments and eye lash extensions. Niccol specializes in handcrafting and formulating skin care products and cosmetics.

She has had a love for skin care since the young age of 9, so it wasn't a surprise when by 11 she was making DIY skincare treatments at home. She didn't want a toy kitchen she wanted a Bunsen burner.

Niccol has clients that travel from all over the world for facials and hair treatments to treat conditions such as alopecia, thinning, early graying, acne, rosacea, dark spots, sensitive reactive red skin, keloids, mole removals and more.

Niccol watched the industry change and frowned on new unhealthy fly by treatment fads. In 2023 she decided to expand by making Pretti Please Beauty Co.'s products available for global sale. She still hand crafts and formulates to ensure the quality of all products. "Skin is like fingerprints everyone's is different". Skin problems can be a result of diet, water intake, work and home environment, medicine, sickness, lifestyle, genes, lack of Self-Care and a plethora or other issues, however the advice in this book can combat a lot of issues when generally applied. Prevention is better than cure. We'll handle the cure too.

This book is not based on trends but products that have been proven to cure and aide in glowing skin, reverse the signs of aging and solutions that provide long term positive results.

Niccol decided to write this book after realizing many of her clients had the same questions. She wanted to help as many people as possible and put all the answers and advice in one place. This book is fun, interactive and has a great read. Niccol runs her skincare company with the aspirations of being the "Berkshire Hathaway of Skin Care". Stay tuned Pretti there is a lot to come.

Stay up to date with Niccol A on Instagram
@NiccolAGordon

APPENDIX: ADDITIONAL RESOURCES

As the founder of "Pretti Please Beauty Co." and editor of "Skincare Starts with Self-care," I'm thrilled to provide you with additional resources to support your transformative journey to nurture both your skin and soul. Below, you'll find valuable resources to enhance your understanding of skincare, self-care, and holistic well-being:

1. Glossary of Skincare Terms:

Navigate the world of skincare with confidence by familiarizing yourself with key terminology. Our glossary provides definitions and explanations for common skincare terms, ensuring you're well-equipped to make informed decisions about your skincare routine.

2. Recommended Reading:

Expand your knowledge and deepen your understanding of skincare, self-care, and holistic wellness with our curated list of recommended reading. From expert skincare guides to inspirational self-care books, these resources offer invaluable insights and practical tips to elevate your beauty and wellness journey.

3. Skincare Product Recommendations:

Discover the perfect skincare products to complement your self-care routine with our curated list of recommendations. From cleansers and moisturizers to serums and masks, each product is carefully selected to nourish your skin and enhance your well-being.

With "Pretti Please Beauty Co.," embark on a transformative journey to nurture your skin and soul and discover the beauty of holistic self-care. Whether you're seeking skincare advice, self-care inspiration, or product recommendations, we're here to support you every step of the way.

Happy reading and glowing,

NICCOL A

EDITOR, "Skincare Starts With Self-Care"

SKIN CARE GLOSSARY / TERMINOLOGY

Acne: a common skin condition characterized by the presence of pimples, blackheads, and whiteheads, often caused by clogged pores, bacteria, and hormonal fluctuations.

Antimicrobial: Ingredients that help kill or inhibit the growth of bacteria, fungi, and other microorganisms on the skin, reducing the risk of infections and breakouts.

Antioxidants: compounds that help protect the skin from damage caused by free radicals, unstable molecules that can lead to premature aging and skin damage.

Alpha Hydroxy Acids (AHAs): Chemical exfoliants that help remove dead skin cells, improve skin texture, and reduce the appearance of fine lines and wrinkles.

Barrier Function: The skin's natural protective barrier, composed of lipids, ceramides, and other substances, that prevents moisture loss and protects against environmental damage.

Beta Hydroxy Acid (BHA): A chemical exfoliant, such as salicylic acid, that penetrates deep into the pores to unclog them and treat acne and blackheads.

Cleanser: a skincare product designed to remove dirt, oil, makeup, and impurities from the skin, leaving it clean and refreshed.

Ceramides: Lipids that help maintain the skin's barrier function, preventing moisture loss and protecting against environmental damage.

Emollients: Ingredients that help soften and smooth the skin by forming a protective barrier to lock in moisture.

Essence: A lightweight, watery skincare product that hydrates, soothes, and prepares the skin to better absorb subsequent skincare products.

Essential Oils: Concentrated plant extracts that provide various benefits to the skin, including hydration, soothing, and antioxidant protection.

Exfoliation: the process of removing dead skin cells from the surface of the skin, promoting cell turnover and revealing smoother, brighter skin underneath.

Humectants: Ingredients that attract moisture from the air and bind it to the skin, helping to keep it hydrated and plump.

Hyaluronic acid: a naturally occurring substance in the skin that helps maintain moisture levels, keeping the skin hydrated, plump, and youthful.

Moisturizer: a skincare product that helps hydrate and nourish the skin, providing essential moisture to maintain a healthy skin barrier.

Niacin-amide: Also known as vitamin B3, niacin-amide helps regulate oil production, improve skin texture, and reduce inflammation and redness.

Peptides: Chains of amino acids that help stimulate collagen production, improve skin firmness and elasticity, and reduce the appearance of wrinkles.

Retinol: a derivative of vitamin a that helps improve the appearance of fine lines, wrinkles, and uneven skin tone by stimulating collagen production and increasing cell turnover.

Serums: a lightweight skincare product with a high concentration of active ingredients, designed to target specific skin concerns such as aging, hydration, or brightening.

Sheet Masks: Single-use face masks made of cloth or paper soaked in serum, designed to deliver concentrated doses of active ingredients to the skin.

SPF: Sun protection factor, a measure of how well a sunscreen protects the skin from harmful uv rays. Higher SPF numbers indicate greater protection.

Sunscreen: a skincare product that helps protect the skin from the sun's uv rays, reducing the risk of sunburn, premature aging, and skin cancer.

Toners: a skincare product used after cleansing to remove any remaining traces of dirt, oil, or makeup and help balance the skin's ph levels.

Tretinoin: A prescription-strength retinoid that helps treat acne, reduce the appearance of fine lines and wrinkles, and improve overall skin texture and tone.

These are just a few of the key terms you may encounter on your skincare journey. Understanding these terms can help you make informed decisions about your skincare routine and achieve your skin health goals.

RECOMMENDED READINGS

1. "Pretti please beauty: skincare starts with self care" by Niccol A - This book offers excellent skin care regimens as well as supportive self care techniques.

2. "The little book of skin care: Korean beauty secrets for healthy, glowing skin" by charlotte cho - discover the secrets of Korean skincare and learn how to achieve radiant, youthful skin with this comprehensive guide.

3. "Skin cleanse: the simple, all-natural program for clear, calm, happy skin" by Adina Grigore - explore the benefits of natural skincare and learn how to cleanse your skin without harsh chemicals or irritants.

4. "The skincare bible: your no-nonsense guide to great skin" by dr. Anjali Mahto - written by a leading dermatologist, this book offers expert advice on skincare routines, product ingredients, and common skin concerns.

5. "The beauty of dirty skin: the surprising science of looking and feeling radiant from the inside out" by Whitney Bowe, MD - discover the connection between gut health, diet, and skincare, and learn how to achieve glowing skin from the inside out.

6. "The Japanese skincare revolution: how to have the most beautiful skin of your life—at any age" by Chizu Saeki - learn the secrets of Japanese skincare and discover simple, effective techniques for achieving flawless skin at any age.

These recommended readings offer valuable insights and practical tips for achieving healthy, radiant skin from experts in the field of skincare and beauty. Happy reading and may your skincare journey be as enlightening as it is transformative!

SKINCARE PRODUCT RECOMMENDATIONS

As you continue on your journey to radiant skin and holistic well-being, allow me to introduce you to some of the exquisite offerings from Pretti please Beauty Co. Our carefully curated line of skincare products is designed to nourish, rejuvenate, and enhance your natural beauty, all while promoting self-care and self-love.

1. Pretti Revival Serum – Passion Fruit / Pomegranate

Infused with potent antioxidants and hydrating hyaluronic acid, our Radiance Revival Serum works wonders to brighten and rejuvenate tired, dull skin. Say goodbye to fine lines and hello to a luminous, youthful complexion.

2. Pretti Potion Moisturizer

Formulated with nourishing botanicals, oils, butters and skin-loving vitamins, our pretti potion Moisturizer provides deep hydration and long-lasting moisture, leaving your skin soft, supple, and glowing with health.

3. Soothing Sensation Cleansers and Soap Bars:

Gentle yet effective, our Soothing Sensation Cleansers and soap bars gently removes impurities and makeup while soothing and calming sensitive skin. Say hello to a clean, refreshed complexion without the irritation.

4. Velvet Skin Whipped Emulsified Body Scrub

Experience the luxurious sensation of our whipped emulsified Body Scrub, a decadent treat for your skin enriched with nourishing oils, exfoliating particles, and aromatic essences. Gently buff away dry, dull skin to reveal a silky-smooth finish that's irresistibly soft to the touch.

5. Serenity Herbal Bath Teas

Indulge in the ultimate relaxation with our Serenity herbal Bath Teas. Infused with soothing herbs and aromatic botanicals, these bath teas transform your bath into a blissful sanctuary of calm and tranquility, leaving you feeling rejuvenated and refreshed from head to toe.

6. Divine Emulsified Body Butter:

Pamper your skin while you in all day moisture with our Divine body butter. Enriched with nourishing oils and replenishing peptides, this luxurious cream works all-day to hydrate, repair, and renew your skin, so will have visibly smoother, more radiant skin.

Each of our products is lovingly crafted with the finest ingredients and backed by our commitment to quality and efficacy. We invite you to experience the transformative power of pretti beauty co. And embark on a journey to radiant skin and self-care bliss.

INDULGE IN THE LUXURY OF SELF-CARE WITH PRETTI BEAUTY CO., WHERE EVERY PRODUCT IS DESIGNED TO NURTURE YOUR SKIN AND NOURISH YOUR SOUL.

PAPERBACK BONUS:

1.	What are some key takeaways or tips you learned from "Skincare Starts with Self-Care" that you plan to incorporate into your skincare routine?

2.	How has your understanding of skincare principles and practices evolved after reading this book? Were there any myths or misconceptions that were debunked?

3.	Did the book change your perspective on natural versus synthetic skincare ingredients? How do you navigate ingredient lists and product labels differently now?

4.	Were there any DIY skincare recipes or treatments in the book that you're excited to try at home? What ingredients or techniques stood out to you the most?

5.	How does the book address skincare concerns specific to different skin types (e.g., oily, dry, sensitive)? Did you find the advice applicable to your own skin type?

6.	What role does self-care play in the book's approach to skincare? How do you prioritize self-care in your own skincare routine, and do you think it's important for overall skin health?

7.	How does the book address the link between skincare and overall health and well-being? In what ways do you think skincare practices can contribute to or reflect one's overall lifestyle?

8.   What are your thoughts on the environmental impact of skincare products and packaging? Did the book offer any insights or recommendations for more sustainable skincare practices?

9.   How does the book address common skincare concerns such as aging, acne, hyperpigmentation, or sun protection? Did you find the advice practical and evidence-based?

10.   How do you plan to continue educating yourself about skincare beyond reading this book? Are there any specific topics or areas of interest you'd like to explore further?

Share your answers and get answers on Instagram, Tik Tok, Facebook and YouTube on our pages @PrettiPleaseBeauty

LET'S DO THIS TOGETHER!!!

This skincare journal provides a space to track your daily skincare routines and write down your progress, while also including fun facts to keep you engaged and informed about skincare.

Day 1: Morning Routine: Cleanser, Toner, Serum, Moisturizer, Sunscreen

Evening Routine: Cleanser, Exfoliator, Toner, Serum, Moisturizer

Day 2: Morning Routine: Cleanser, Toner, Serum, Eye Cream, Moisturizer, Sunscreen

Evening: Cleanser, Toner, Serum, Moisturizer

Day 3: Morning Routine: Cleanser, Toner, Essence, Serum, Moisturizer

Evening: Double Cleanse, Toner, Serum, Moisturizer

Day 4: Morning Routine: Cleanser, Toner, Serum, Sheet Mask, Moisturizer

Evening: Cleanser, Toner, Serum, Moisturizer

Day 5: Morning Routine: Cleanser, Toner, Serum, Moisturizer, Sunscreen

Evening: Cleanser, Toner, Serum, Moisturizer

Fun Fact: Did you know that the ancient

Egyptians were among the first to practice skincare, using natural ingredients like honey and milk for their beauty rituals?

Day 6: Morning Routine: Cleanser, Toner, Vitamin C, Serum, Moisturizer

Evening Routine: Cleanser, Toner, Serum, Moisturizer

Day 7: Morning Routine: Cleanser, Toner, Hyaluronic Acid, Serum, Moisturizer

Evening: Cleanser, Toner, Serum, Moisturizer

Day 8: Morning Routine: Cleanser, Toner, Essence, Serum, Moisturizer

Evening: Double Cleanse, Toner, Serum, Moisturizer

Day 9: Morning Routine: Cleanser, Exfoliating Scrub, Serum, Moisturizer

Evening: Cleanser, Toner, Serum, Moisturizer

Day 10: Morning Routine: Cleanser, Toner, Serum, Moisturizer, Sunscreen

Evening: Cleanser, Toner, Serum, Moisturizer, Spot Treatment

Fun Fact: The skin is the largest organ in the human body, with an average surface area of about 22 square feet!

Day 11: Morning Routine: Cleanser, Toner, Essence, Serum, Moisturizer

Evening Routine: Cleanser, Toner, Serum, Moisturizer

Day 12: Morning Routine: Cleanser, Toner, Vitamin C, Serum, Moisturizer

Evening: Cleanser, Toner, Serum, Moisturizer

Day 13: Morning Routine: Cleanser, Toner, Hyaluronic Acid, Serum, Moisturizer

Evening: Double Cleanser, Toner, Serum, Moisturizer

Day 14: Morning Routine: Cleanser, Exfoliating Scrub, Serum, Moisturizer

Evening: Cleanser, Toner, Serum, Moisturizer

Day 15: Morning Routine: Cleanser, Toner, Serum, Moisturizer, Sunscreen

Evening: Cleanser, Toner, Serum, Moisturizer, Spot Treatment

84

Fun Fact: Your skin sheds around 30,000 to 40,000 dead skin cells every minute, which adds up to over 9 pounds of dead skin cells every year!

www.ingramcontent.com/pod-product-compliance
Lightning Source LLC
Chambersburg PA
CBHW061253250726
48653CB00002B/646